Herbal Remedies for Weight Loss

Unlocking Nature's Secrets

Jessica Hensley

Table of contents

Chapter 1

Understanding Weight Loss and Herbal Remedies:

Weight loss is a complex process influenced by various factors including diet, physical activity, metabolism, and hormonal balance. While conventional approaches such as calorie restriction and exercise play a significant role in weight management, herbal remedies offer a natural and holistic approach to supporting weight loss goals.

1. Fundamentals of Weight Loss:
Weight loss occurs when the body expends more calories than it consumes, leading to a deficit that prompts the body to burn stored fat for energy. Factors such as age, genetics, metabolism, hormonal balance, and lifestyle

habits influence an individual's ability to lose weight effectively.

2. Herbal Remedies for Weight Loss:
   - Herbal remedies encompass a wide range of plant-based substances known for their medicinal properties and therapeutic effects on the body.
   - Certain herbs contain bioactive compounds that can support weight loss by boosting metabolism, suppressing appetite, increasing fat oxidation, and improving digestion and nutrient absorption.

3. Popular Herbs for Weight Loss:
   - Green Tea: Rich in antioxidants and catechins, green tea boosts metabolism and enhances fat burning, making it a popular ingredient in many weight loss supplements.
   - Garcinia Cambogia: Derived from the fruit rind of the Garcinia cambogia tree, this herb contains hydroxy citric acid (HCA), which may help suppress appetite and inhibit fat production.

- Ginger: Known for its anti-inflammatory and digestive properties, ginger can aid in weight loss by promoting satiety, reducing cravings, and improving digestion.

- Turmeric: Curcumin, the active compound in turmeric, has been shown to support weight loss by reducing inflammation, regulating blood sugar levels, and promoting fat metabolism.

- Cinnamon: This aromatic spice may help regulate blood sugar levels, reduce insulin resistance, and improve metabolic function, contributing to weight loss when incorporated into the diet.

4. Mechanisms of Action:

- Herbal remedies exert their effects through various mechanisms, including thermogenesis, appetite suppression, inhibition of fat absorption, and modulation of metabolic pathways.

- These herbs may also influence hormones such as leptin, ghrelin, insulin, and cortisol, which play key roles in appetite regulation, energy balance, and fat storage.

5. Safety and Considerations:
- While herbal remedies are generally considered safe when used as directed, it's essential to consult with a healthcare professional before incorporating them into your weight loss regimen, especially if you have underlying health conditions or are taking medications.
- Some herbs may interact with medications or have contraindications for certain populations, so it's crucial to be informed and cautious.

Understanding weight loss and the role of herbal remedies can empower individuals to make informed decisions about their health and explore natural approaches to achieving their weight loss goals. By combining herbal remedies with a balanced diet, regular exercise, and healthy lifestyle habits, individuals can optimize their chances of success on their weight loss journey.

Explaining the Fundamentals of Weight Loss: Calories, Metabolism, and Body Composition

1. Calories:
   - Calories are units of energy derived from the foods and beverages we consume.
   - The body requires a certain amount of calories to perform basic functions such as breathing, circulating blood, and maintaining body temperature.
   - When we consume more calories than our body needs for these functions, the excess calories are stored as fat, leading to weight gain.
   - Conversely, when we consume fewer calories than our body needs, the body taps into its fat stores to make up for the energy deficit, leading to weight loss.

2. Metabolism:

- Metabolism refers to the complex series of chemical reactions that occur within the body to convert food into energy.

- Basal metabolic rate (BMR) is the number of calories the body needs at rest to maintain vital functions.

- Factors such as age, gender, genetics, muscle mass, and hormone levels influence individual metabolic rates.

- People with higher metabolic rates tend to burn more calories at rest and during physical activity, making it easier for them to lose weight or maintain a healthy weight.

3. Body Composition:

- Body composition refers to the proportion of fat, muscle, bone, and water in the body.

- Two individuals with the same weight can have different body compositions, with one having a higher percentage of lean muscle mass and the other having more body fat.

- Lean muscle tissue is metabolically active and burns more calories at rest than fat tissue, contributing to a higher metabolic rate.

- Body composition plays a significant role in determining overall health and metabolic efficiency.

4. Weight Loss Process:

- To lose weight, individuals need to create a calorie deficit by consuming fewer calories than they expend.

- This can be achieved through a combination of dietary changes, increased physical activity, and lifestyle modifications.

- A safe and sustainable rate of weight loss is generally considered to be 0.5 to 2 pounds per week.

- Gradual weight loss allows for the preservation of lean muscle mass and helps prevent metabolic slowdown.

5. Factors Influencing Weight Loss:

- While calorie intake and expenditure are primary determinants of weight loss, other factors also play a role, including genetics, hormonal imbalances, medication use, sleep quality, stress levels, and environmental factors.

- It's essential to adopt a holistic approach to weight loss that addresses these factors and promotes overall health and well-being.

Understanding the fundamentals of weight loss, including calories, metabolism, and body composition, empowers individuals to make informed decisions about their dietary and lifestyle choices. By creating a calorie deficit through healthy eating habits and regular physical activity, individuals can achieve sustainable weight loss and improve their overall health and fitness levels.

Discussing the Benefits and Limitations of Herbal Remedies Compared to Conventional Weight Loss Methods:

1. Benefits of Herbal Remedies:

a. Natural Ingredients: Herbal remedies for weight loss are derived from plants and botanical sources, making them natural and often well-tolerated by the body.

b. Fewer Side Effects: Compared to some conventional weight loss medications, herbal remedies typically have fewer side effects and are less likely to cause adverse reactions.

c. Holistic Approach: Herbal remedies often take a holistic approach to weight loss, addressing not only physical factors but also emotional and mental aspects of health.

d. Supporting Metabolism: Certain herbs may help support metabolism, enhance fat burning, and promote overall energy levels, contributing to more effective weight loss over time.

e. Nutritional Support: Many herbal remedies contain vitamins, minerals, and antioxidants that support overall health and well-being, providing additional nutritional benefits beyond weight loss.

2. Limitations of Herbal Remedies:

a. Limited Scientific Evidence: While some herbal remedies have shown promising results in preliminary studies, the scientific evidence supporting their effectiveness for weight loss is often limited or inconclusive.

b. Variable Quality and Potency: The quality and potency of herbal supplements can vary widely between brands and manufacturers, making it challenging to ensure consistency and efficacy.

c. Slow Results: Herbal remedies may take longer to produce noticeable weight loss results compared to conventional weight loss methods such as prescription medications or surgical interventions.

d. Individual Variability: The effectiveness of herbal remedies for weight loss can vary significantly between individuals, depending on factors such as genetics, lifestyle, and overall health status.

e. Lack of Regulation: Herbal supplements are not subject to the same rigorous regulatory standards as pharmaceutical drugs, leading to concerns about product safety, purity, and accuracy of labeling.

3. Comparison to Conventional Weight Loss Methods:

a. Conventional Methods: Conventional weight loss methods, such as calorie restriction, exercise, and behavioral modifications, are often supported by robust scientific evidence and clinical research.

b. Faster Results: Conventional weight loss methods may produce more rapid and predictable results compared to herbal remedies, making them appealing for individuals seeking immediate weight loss outcomes.

c. Medical Supervision: Some conventional weight loss methods, such as prescription medications or bariatric surgery, require medical supervision and oversight to ensure safety and efficacy.

d. Complementary Approach: Herbal remedies can complement conventional weight loss methods by providing additional support for metabolism, appetite control, and overall well-being.

Herbal remedies offer natural alternatives for weight loss that may be appealing to individuals seeking holistic approaches to health and wellness. While herbal remedies have several potential benefits, they also have limitations and may not be suitable for everyone. Individuals need to weigh the potential risks and benefits of herbal remedies carefully and consult with healthcare professionals before incorporating them into their weight loss regimen. Additionally, herbal remedies can be used as part of a comprehensive approach to weight loss that includes healthy eating, regular physical activity, and lifestyle modifications.

Chapter 2

Powerful Herbs For Weight Loss And Their Benefits

A few spices and flavors might assist with supporting weight reduction notwithstanding a nutritious eating regimen and customary actual work. This can incorporate cayenne pepper and cinnamon, among others.
It's a well-known fact that what you're putting on your plate assumes a focal part in weight reduction.

Yet, what you keep in your flavor bureau might be comparably significant.
Numerous spices and flavors have been displayed to battle desires and lift fat consumption and weight reduction.
Once in a while, the key to weight reduction might lie in the most unforeseen of spots.

At the point when the food is dull, it tends to be challenging to adhere to an eating regimen. Fortunately, spices and flavors can give flavor while likewise aiding the decrease of unhealthy food desires. There are numerous spices for weight reduction that you can browse. These spices offer mitigating, cancer prevention agents, are hostile to diabetes, cholesterol-bringing down, and chemical adjusting properties and help in weight reduction. To assist you with getting in shape naturally, attempt these 16 brilliant spices. Continue to peruse to know more.

Best Spices For Weight Reduction

1. Cinnamon For Weight reduction

Cinnamon is demonstrated to assist with decreasing weight and battling stoutness. It assists with supporting digestion, manages glucose, and assumes an essential part in bringing down LDL cholesterol and triglycerides. With its advantages, it turns into an optimal sauce for those with diabetes.

Instructions to Consume Cinnamon For Weight Reduction

You can take 1 ½ - 1 teaspoon of powdered cinnamon or 1 cinnamon bark absorbed water for the time being. Drink cinnamon-mixed water first thing consistently for quite some time to obtain the ideal outcomes.

Cinnamon Tea Recipe

Fixings

• 1 ½ teaspoon cinnamon powder

• 1 cup water

Instructions to Plan

• Carry some water to bubble.

• Add the cinnamon powder and let the water bubble for 2-3 minutes more.

• Strain the cinnamon tea before drinking.

Benefits

Cinnamon smothers cravings brings down awful cholesterol, and speeds up the metabolic rate. The warm water assists flush out every one of the poisons and supports bettering solid discharge. It additionally forestalls bulging.

2. Fenugreek For Weight reduction

Fenugreek seeds are demonstrated to treat metabolic dysfunctions. Fenugreek seed-remove supplementation lessens dietary fat utilization. The seeds additionally assist with decreasing cholesterol, work on fat assimilation, and improve insulin responsiveness.

The most effective method to Consume Fenugreek For Weight reduction

Require 1 teaspoon of fenugreek seeds each day with 1 cup of water. You may likewise crush the fenugreek seeds, store them in a perfect container, and use them in curries, dal soup, or smoothies.

Fenugreek Seeds Weight Reduction Recipe

Fixings

• 1 teaspoon of fenugreek seeds

• 1 cup of water

Instructions to Plan

• Drench 1 teaspoon of fenugreek seeds in some water for the time being.

• Polish off the water as well as seeds both first thing on the void stomach.

Benefits

It supports digestion, forestalls weight set off by pressure and aggravation, flushes out poisons from the colon, and diminishes the gamble of insulin opposition regularly tracked down in ladies with PCOS.

3. Garlic For Weight reduction

The dynamic fixing in garlic, allicin, helps treat cardiovascular circumstances, metabolic issues, and high glucose. It likewise has hostile to growth properties and assists with supporting resistance. A logical report affirms that garlic supports digestion, assists with decreasing fat testimony, and may assist in diminishing with bodying weight.

The most effective method to Consume Garlic For Weight reduction

You can have one clove of garlic consistently for the best outcomes. You can likewise remember garlic for your day-to-day recipes to add taste and flavour. Truth be told, Indian cooking is inadequate without the digestion supporting garlic and the oil separated from mustard seeds.

Garlic Weight Reduction Recipe

Fixings

• 1 clove garlic

• 1 cup water

• Juice of ½ a lime

Instructions to Plan

• Utilize a mortar and pestle to squash the garlic clove.

• Add it to some water.

• Add lime juice, mix well, and drink in one go.

Benefits

The lime juice helps cut the impactful smell and taste of the garlic. Limes are additionally plentiful in L-ascorbic acid. L-ascorbic acid may likewise advance weight reduction, however, more exploration is required in such a manner. Garlic helps lower cholesterol, further develops heart well-being, has hostile to disease properties, and helps weight reduction by keeping your food cravings under control.

4. Hibiscus For Weight reduction

Hibiscus tea, the vermillion-shaded hibiscus blossom separate, helps in weight reduction. A few examinations have shown that hibiscus separate is a craving suppressant that diminishes stomach weight, decreases the gamble of the non-alcoholic greasy liver, fat collection, adipogenesis, and lessens hunger chemicals, ghrelin and pulse. Hibiscus utilization as tea prompts amazing thinning impacts.

Instructions to Take Hibiscus Tea For Weight Reduction

One cup of hibiscus tea contains around 1.5 grams of hibiscus calyx. You can have up to 2 cups of hibiscus tea each day.

Hibiscus Tea Weight Reduction Recipe

Fixings

• 1teaspoons dried hibiscus blossoms

• 2 cups water

• 1 teaspoon honey

The most effective method to Get ready

• Put the dried hibiscus blossoms into a tea kettle.

• Bubble 2 cups of water and fill the tea kettle.

• Allow it to soak for 5-6 minutes.

• Strain some hibiscus tea.

• Add honey and mix well.

Benefits

Hibiscus tea forestalls disturbance in the stomach has diuretic properties, may help in bringing down cholesterol, and further develops solid discharge. Honey is valuable against throat diseases and has antimicrobial, cancer prevention agents, calming, resistance helping, and hostile to growth properties. In any case, further exploration is expected to affirm overabundance utilization of hibiscus tea that can be consumed in a day with next to no consequences for pulse.

5. Green Tea For Weight reduction

Green tea is rich in cancer prevention agents called catechins. One of the catechins, epigallocatechin gallate, is a digestion sponsor. Likewise, green tea contains some caffeine that invigorates fat consumption and better muscle execution. Green tea is experimentally demonstrated to stifle hunger check desires, and animate chemicals that assist with consuming fat.

The most effective method to Take Green Tea For Weight reduction

It is best you utilize the green tea leaves to set up some tea. You can have upwards of 3 cups of green tea each day. You might drink some green tea 20-30 minutes before dinner.

Green Tea Weight Reduction Recipe

Fixings

• 1 teaspoon green tea leaves

• 1 cup water

• ¼ teaspoon cinnamon

Step-by-step instructions to Get ready

• Carry some water to bubble.

• Add the cinnamon powder and stew for 2 minutes.

• Switch the fire off and add the green tea leaves.

• Allow them to soak for 5-7 minutes.

• Strain and mix for a long time before drinking. The following are two alternate ways of getting ready for green tea.

Benefits

Green tea and cinnamon are strong weight reduction specialists. Green tea supports digestion and assists with softening fat. Cinnamon helps weight reduction by directing glucose levels and insulin levels, bringing down cholesterol, and smothering cravings.

6. Dark Pepper For Weight reduction

Dark pepper is wealthy in piperine. Piperine gives dark pepper its trademark flavour and represses the making of fat cells (adipogenesis). Subsequently, consuming dark pepper helps to lessen weight. Pepper additionally has cancer prevention agents, calming, hostile to microbial, stomach capability improving, and energizer properties.

Step-by-step instructions to Consume Dark Pepper For Weight reduction

You can either bite 5 dark peppercorns each day or add them to your juice or food recipes.

Dark Pepper Weight Reduction Recipe

Fixings

• ¼ teaspoon newly ground dark pepper

• ½ teaspoon honey

• 1 cup warm water

Instructions to Plan

• Add 1 teaspoon honey and ¼ teaspoon dark pepper to some warm water.

• Mix a long time before drinking.

Benefits

Dark pepper helps weight reduction by forestalling fat cell blend and honey aides support invulnerability and keep a solid stomach. This beverage with dark pepper and honey aids flush out the poisons from your body.

7. Ginger For Weight reduction

Ginger assists support digestion, increments with fatting cell breakdown, represses fat assimilation, and assists with checking extreme craving. Ginger water likewise decreases body weight, midsection to-hip proportion, fasting glucose, and insulin opposition file.

Instructions to Consume Ginger For Weight Reduction

You can bite ½ inch of ginger root or add it to your juice, smoothies, or food recipes. You can likewise make ginger water by heating some water with 1-inch ginger root. Drinking it chills me off.

Ginger Tea Weight Reduction Recipe

Fixings

• ½ inch ginger

• 1 teaspoon honey

• 1 cup water

The most effective method to Plan

• Carry some water to bubble.

• Utilize a mortar and pestle to squash the ginger root.

• Add the squashed ginger root to the bubbling water.

• Allow it to bubble for 2 minutes more.

• Switch off the fire and add honey.

• Strain and mix for a long time before drinking.

Benefits

Ginger works on gastrointestinal and liver well-being, flushes out poisons, forestalls throat diseases, and assists soften with fatting. Honey adjusts areas of strength for the ginger, adds to the pleasantness of the beverage, and lifts the resistant framework.

8. Turmeric For Weight reduction

Turmeric contains curcumin that helps lower awful cholesterol and irritation to assist with decreasing weight. Curcumin consumption in individuals with metabolic disorders was found to assist with decreasing BMI, body weight, midsection periphery, and expanded adiponectin (a peptide that invigorates unsaturated fat oxidation, insulin responsiveness, and increments calorie use).

The most effective method to Consume Turmeric For Weight reduction

Bite ½ an inch of turmeric root or ½ to 1 teaspoon of turmeric powder each day.

Turmeric Weight Reduction Recipe

Fixings

• ½ inch turmeric root

- 1 cup warm water

- ½ lime juice

The most effective method to Plan

- Utilize a mortar and pestle to smash the turmeric root.

- Add it to some warm water.

- Add lime juice.

- Mix for a long time before drinking.

Benefits

It might advance weight reduction and further develop stomach wellbeing. It likewise forestalls microbial contaminations, mends wounds, and assists with diminishing the force of torment.

9. Cardamom For Weight reduction

Concentrates on saying that cardamom has cell reinforcement and mitigating properties that might end up being useful to increment insulin responsiveness and decrease all-out cholesterol in overweight and hefty ladies with prediabetes. It might likewise assist with working on the grade of greasy liver in individuals with non-alcoholic greasy liver sickness. You can either utilize green or dark cardamon. In any case, recounted proof recommends consuming dark cardamom for weight reduction.

The most effective method to Consume Cardamom For Weight reduction

You can take ½ a teaspoon of dark cardamom powder one time each day.

Cardamom Weight Reduction Recipe

Fixings

- ½ teaspoon dark cardamom powder

- 1 cup water

- 1 teaspoon green tea leaves

Step by Step-by-step Instructions to Plan

- Carry some water to bubble.

- Add cardamom powder and let it bubble for 2 minutes more.

- Switch off the fire and add green tea leaves.

- Allow them to soak for 5 minutes.

- Strain the tea and mix for a long time before drinking.

Benefits

Green tea is a digestion promoter and helps flush out poisons. Cardamom expands the interior internal heat level and may assist with softening out the additional muscle versus fat.

10. Cayenne Pepper For Weight reduction
Cayenne pepper is one of the fixings in Beyonce's renowned expert scrub eating routine. It is rich in capsaicin, which animates the body to consume fat and has detoxifying impacts on the body. Adding cayenne pepper to your food in restricted sums can assist with decreasing cravings by expanding satiety. It contains thermogenic intensities that likewise increment fat digestion and thermogenesis, and restrain the development of fat cells.

Instructions to Consume Cayenne Pepper For Weight Reduction

Take ¼ teaspoon of cayenne pepper with your juice or smoothie two times every day.

Cayenne Pepper Weight Reduction Recipe

Fixings

• ¼ teaspoon cayenne pepper

• 1 lime

• 1 cup water

The most effective method to Get ready

• Get out the juice of a lime into a glass.

• Add some water and ¼ teaspoon of cayenne pepper.

• Mix for a long time before drinking.

Benefits

The hotness of cayenne pepper is impeccably adjusted by the lime's acidic taste. The two fixings might help weight reduction by supporting digestion and consuming muscle versus fat.

11. Cumin For Weight reduction

Cumin or jeera is one more famous zest that is utilized in numerous foods across the world. Cumin seeds assist with further developing processing and have cell reinforcement, against inflammatory, hostile to the microbial enemy of hypertensive, antihistamines, hypoglycemic, malignant growth, and insusceptibility supporting properties. An investigation discovered that cumin powder might assist with decreasing BMI, midriff circuit, serum fatty substances, terrible cholesterol, and muscle versus fat ratio.

The most effective method to Consume Cumin For Weight reduction

Take 1 teaspoon of cumin seeds absorbed water or add ½ teaspoon of cumin seed powder in juices or food recipes.

Cumin Weight Reduction Recipe

Fixings

• 1 teaspoon cumin seeds

• 1 cup water

• ½ teaspoon honey powder

Step by Step-by-step Instructions to Plan

• Douse the cumin seeds in water for the time being.

• Heat the water till it turns out to be warm.

• Strain the water and add honey.

• Mix a long time before drinking.

Benefits

Cumin seeds are very useful in keeping up with stomach wellbeing. It likewise assists one lay down with bettering and lessens the gamble of respiratory issues, normal colds, sickliness, and skin problems. Honey is an antibacterial specialist and helps flush out poisons.

12. Rosemary For Weight reduction

Rosemary has cell reinforcement and antimicrobial properties. It likewise decreases blood glucose levels and cholesterol by expanding liver glycolysis (breakdown of glucose units put away in the liver) and fat oxidation.

Step-by-step instructions to Consume Rosemary For Weight reduction

You can require 400 mg of rosemary tablets threefold every day. You can likewise involve new or dried rosemary in food.

Rosemary Weight Reduction Recipe

Fixings

• 1 teaspoon new rosemary

• 1 cup water

The most effective method to Get ready

• Carry some water to bubble.

• Switch the fire off and add rosemary.

• Allow it to soak for 5-7 minutes.

• Strain and drink.

Benefits

Rosemary lessens glucose and cholesterol. It likewise helps flush out the poisons from the colon and forestalls bulging. Other remedial and weight-reduction spices that you might attempt are parsley, coriander, oregano, basil, thyme, liquorice root, garcinia cambogia, and sage.

13. Aloe Vera For Weight reduction

Aloe vera is known for its purgative properties in Ayurveda. It likewise lessens aggravation and helps the treatment of stomach issues and type 2 diabetes. Aloe vera likewise decreases body weight, muscle-to-fat ratio mass, and insulin opposition in individuals with prediabetes.

Instructions to Consume Aloe Vera For Weight Reduction

You can take 1-2 teaspoons of aloe vera and remove it consistently. Or on the other hand, you can scoop out the aloe vera gel from the leaf and blend it in with your morning juice or smoothie.

Aloe Vera Weight Reduction Recipe

Fixings

• 1 teaspoon aloe vera gel

• 1 cup water

Step by Step-by-step Instructions to Plan

• Pound the aloe vera gel utilizing the rear of a spoon.

• Add water and mix well.

Benefits

Drinking this water each day will keep your skin and hair solid. It will likewise keep your stomach-related framework solid and may advance faster weight reduction.

14. Dandelion For Weight reduction

Dandelions are delightful, and they are palatable! A logical survey distributed in The Audit of Diabetic Examinations affirms that dandelions are hostile to diabetes, hostile to stoutness, and calming, hyperglycemic, and cell reinforcement properties. It likewise increments insulin awareness and insulin emission and further develops assimilation. Dandelion leaves may likewise assist with lessening serum glucose, fatty oil, and cholesterol levels.

Step-by-step instructions to Consume Dandelion For Weight reduction

You can take 1-2 teaspoons of dandelion or 1 dandelion pill with a full glass of water.

Dandelion Weight Reduction Recipe

Fixings

• 1 teaspoon dandelion

• 1 cup water

Step-by-step instructions to Get ready

• Carry some water to bubble.

• Add the dandelion and let it bubble for 2-3 minutes.

• Strain and let it cool for a couple of moments before drinking.

Benefits

Dandelions are wealthy in fibre and may assist with forestalling the retention of fat particles. The cell reinforcements assist with searching the unsafe oxygen revolutionaries and flush out the poisons. Other cell reinforcement-rich spices to go after weight reduction are cilantro, chamomile, straight leaf, lavender, lemon salve, passionflower, valerian root, and passionflower.

15. Ginseng For Weight reduction

Ginseng has been utilized as a medication by the Chinese for quite a long time. It diminishes irritation and stress, smothers hunger, diminishes glucose ingestion and lipid digestion, lessens insulin obstruction and the gamble of liver harm, brings down LDL cholesterol, and directs glucose levels. Stress, unregulated glucose, and elevated cholesterol are supporters of terrible well-being and weight gain. A concentration on Korean ladies affirms that ginseng is a viable homegrown solution for weight reduction.

Instructions to Consume Ginseng For Weight Reduction

Require 5 gm of ginseng removed two times every day. You can diminish the sum to 2 gm following fourteen days. You can likewise add 15-25 drops of ginseng extricate in your tea or water two times every day.

Ginseng Tea Weight Reduction Recipe

Fixings

• 1 teaspoon of ginseng extricate

• 500 mL water

• 1 tablespoon of lime juice

• A touch of cinnamon powder

• 1 tablespoon of lime juice

• A spot of cinnamon powder

Step by Step-by-step Instructions to Plan

• Bubble water in a skillet and let it cool for 5 minutes.

• Add the ginseng concentrate and let it steep for 5 minutes.

• Strain the water and add lime juice and cinnamon powder.

• Mix for a long time before drinking.

Benefits

Ginseng concentrate will assist you with unwinding, support your energy levels and metabolic rate, and lower cholesterol, and direct glucose levels. Cinnamon additionally helps weight reduction by bringing down terrible cholesterol levels and circulatory strain. Lime is a storage facility of L-ascorbic acid that helps support resistance.

16. Inlet Leaves For Weight reduction

Episodic proof recommends that the rich fiber content in narrow leaves might help digestion and keep your stomach full, which might support solid weight the executives.

Benefits

Research recommends that narrowed leaves assist with expanding high-thickness lipoprotein cholesterol (HDL) and reduction of low-thickness cholesterol (LDL) levels in individuals with diabetes. Since corpulence and diabetes are connected to higher LDL cholesterol levels, consuming narrow leaves might support weight reduction.

Note: With regards to homegrown activities for weight reduction, it is essential to comprehend that utilizing spices alone won't bring about extensive or enduring weight reduction.

Besides these spices, there are a few different ones that are as of now being scrutinized.

17. Green Espresso Bean Concentrate

Green espresso bean separation is generally found in many weight reduction supplements.
It's produced using espresso beans that haven't been broiled and are high in chlorogenic corrosive, which is remembered to represent its potential weight-bringing down impacts.
One investigation discovered that consuming green espresso decreased weight file (BMI) and gut fat in 20 members, even without any progressions in calorie consumption.
Overall. In any case, analysts noticed that the quality and size of accessible examinations were fairly restricted.

Hence, more excellent examinations are expected to assess the adequacy of green espresso beans on weight reduction.
Rundown Green espresso bean
separation is produced using unroasted espresso beans. Some examination proposes that it
could assist with diminishing body weight and paunch fat.

Green Espresso Bean Concentrate Advantages

1. May Assist With Weight or Fat Misfortune

2. Can Assist with normalizing Glucose

3. May Assist with bringing down Circulatory strain

4. Has Against Maturing Impacts Due to Containing Cell reinforcements

5. Can Assist with further developing Energy Levels

6. Can Help You Concentration and Work on Your Mindset

18. Caralluma Fimbriata

Caralluma Fimbriata is a spice that is much of the time remembered for some eating routine pills.
It's remembered to work by expanding levels of serotonin, a synapse that straightforwardly influences craving.
One 12-week concentration in 33 individuals found that members who took Caralluma Fimbriata had fundamentally more noteworthy reductions in midsection fat and body weight, contrasted with those on a fake treatment.
Another little review showed that consuming 1 gram of Caralluma Fimbriata every day for quite some time prompted

decreases in weight and craving levels, contrasted with a benchmark group.

Synopsis Caralluma
Fimbriata is a spice generally utilized in diet pills that might be useful to diminish hunger to invigorate weight reduction.

Likely Advantages

1. Smothers Craving

The most notable expected advantage of Caralluma Fimbriata is its craving stifling impacts. It's accepted to significantly affect the piece of the mind that directs craving control.

2. May Battle Stoutness

C. fimbriata is utilized in conventional medication to battle corpulence since it fills in as a characteristic craving suppressant. The delicious is remembered to impede the impacts of specific catalysts that assume a part in fat development. This powers the body to consume fat stores all things being equal, possibly prompting weight reduction.

3. May Improve Perseverance

C. fimbriata is known for its capacity to upgrade perseverance, albeit this advantage has not been demonstrated with research. Some concentrates consolidate Baramulla fimbriata extricates with a weight-lessening diet and active work. Members in these examinations have shown decreased midsection boundaries.

Chapter 3

Natural Home Remedies To Reduce Belly Fat

Reducing stomach fat is something many individuals want. It may very well be a direct result of that shirt or dress that doesn't fit or out of the humiliation of having a swelling stomach. However, paunch fat can present more serious well-being gambles with diabetes, weight, and heart diseases.[1] Anything the explanation might be, decreasing tummy fat is turning into a significant wellness objective for individuals.

Gut fat is the collection of fats in the midsection. It is likewise called instinctive fat, which is more normal in men. Doing activity and following a sound eating regimen is a successful and effective method for controlling gut fat.[1] There are explicit cures that you can use at home to assist you with decreasing midsection fat and partake in a better and fitter life.

What Causes Gut Fat?

The things that can cause fat aggregation in your body are:

• Absence of actual activity

• Abuse of liquor

• Eating more than whatever is required

A few different variables can likewise prompt fat gathering in the body:

• Hypothyroidism (underactive thyroid organ)

• Taking antidepressants, antipsychotics, or anti-conception medication pills

• Pregnancy

• Menopause

• Stress

• Disturbed rest

• Stopping smoking2

Cholesterol amalgamation happens during the night in our body. A calorie-shortage diet and early supper, as a rule before 7 pm, assist a ton in diminishing stomach fattening. Different measures like ordinary activity and great rest are similarly significant.

Side effects of Paunch Fat:

Side effects of paunch fat include:

• Extreme fat collection in the stomach

• An expanded waistline than before is likewise a decent mark of stomach fat.

Expanded paunch fat can prompt corpulence in individuals. Corpulence can expand the gamble of different circumstances like diabetes, heart illnesses, stroke, hypertension, sickness of the gallbladder, stroke, joint pain, kidney sickness, greasy liver sickness, rest apnea, disease, and issues in pregnancy.

Home Solutions for Stomach Fat:

Gone are the days when individuals acknowledged stomach fat as a standard difference in maturing. All things considered, individuals are turning out to be more mindful and need to have a solid body. Here are a few home cures that could assist with losing gut fat.

1. Bean stew Pepper:

Admission of capsicum or stew pepper might be connected with the decrease of gathered fat in the body. Additionally, capsicum may be important to advance the utilization of fat gathered in the body.5 You can place capsicum in your food sources and vegetable dishes to assist in lessening fattening in the gut.

2. Ginger:

Ginger might offer numerous medical advantages for individuals needing to diminish stomach fat. Taking ginger is related to improved fat digestion in the body. Ginger could likewise work with the use of fat in the body. Taking ginger likewise lessens fat capacity in the body, causing a general decrease in body weight.5

3. Turmeric:

Turmeric has numerous well-being benefits. Turmeric might decrease the fat stored in the body. It could assist with lessening muscle-to-fat ratio and body weight according to creature studies.5 You can blend a few turmeric in a glass of warm water and take it each day to decrease midsection fat.

4. Cumin:

Cumin or jeera is a typical seed utilized as a flavor in numerous Indian families. Cumin has numerous medical advantages and is frequently utilized for managing runs and other stomach illnesses. What's more, admission of cumin might assist with improving fat breakdown in the body and diminish the appetite.6 These advantages of cumin could assist you with lessening stomach fat and accomplishing a solid weight yourself. You can place cumin in different food varieties, dishes and mixed greens.

Midsection fat, generally known as instinctive fat, is an early mark of coronary illness, stroke, diabetes and sudden passing. Getting it completely checked by a doctor is of most extreme significance to forestall long-haul confusion.

5. Lemon:

Lemon is significant for well-being in the forestalling way of life-related illnesses. For instance, lemon advances fat digestion and diminishes body weight and fat accumulation.7 Lemon could assist with decreasing the aggregation of stomach fat. Add lemon juice to a glass of warm water and savor it in the morning while starving.

6. Green Tea:

Green tea is a well-known drink used to keep up with well-being and is useful in forestalling various illnesses. Green tea admission could diminish fat amassing, according to a few creature studies. Different advantages like a decrease in body weight and greasy tissues have additionally been observed.8 Blend some green tea and drink it each day to assist with diminishing paunch fat and oversaw weight.

7. Work out:

Doing a moderate measure of actual activity might assist with combating stomach fat. You can begin by completing 30 minutes of activity every day to assist with overseeing midsection fat and diminishing weight. You can gradually expand your activity term. Practicing with loads (strength preparation) is a successful method for overseeing stomach fat. Another successful activity is sit-ups (spot workouts).

8. Sound Eating regimen:

Diet is a significant component overseeing the collection of fat in the body. What you eat and the piece size matter, and you ought to give close consideration to it. Make vegetables, natural products, and whole grains a piece of your ordinary eating regimen. Keep away from straightforward starches like white bread, sweet beverages, and refined grains.1 Here are some great dietary patterns that you can follow for a solid living:

• Ensure your eating routine contains an adequate number of nutrients and minerals for sound living.

• Try not to start eating better (under 1100 calories every day), as it's undependable, and there is no proof to help that it works.

• Find out about alternate ways of overseeing pressure other than incessant nibbling, like reflection or yoga.

• Pursue good food decisions at home as well as in eateries.

• Pick better nibbling choices.

• Peruse the nourishment names at the back when you search for groceries.2

Making appropriate eating routine changes and changing dietary patterns is a successful method for diminishing stomach fat.

However, some concentrates show the advantages of the given spices and home solutions for managing stomach fat, but these are deficient. There is a requirement for additional investigations to lay out the genuine degree of the advantages of these spices and home cures on human well-being. In this manner, these ought to be taken with alertness and never as a substitute for clinical treatment.

Trans fats found in cakes, rolls, hard margarine, action items, baked goods, pies and broiled food varieties are fiery and make insulin opposition in the body, which is the way gut fat aggregates without any problem. Avoiding these foods is better.

Wellbeing Of Spices For Weight reduction

Spices are perfect for weight reduction and for adding flavor to food. Be that as it may, don't consume such a large number of the spices referenced previously. Additionally, be cautious about any hypersensitive responses. Take extraordinary consideration assuming you are now under clinical treatment for heftiness, diabetes, stomach sickness, or coronary illness. Assuming you have quite recently conceived an offspring or are pregnant, try not to bring any new food into your eating regimen without talking with your primary care physician.

End

Fat collection in the tummy can make individuals humiliated and increase the gamble of numerous unfavourable ailments like diabetes and corpulence. On account of these reasons, individuals need to decrease their midsection fat. The absence of actual activity and indulging are a portion of the explanations behind expanded midsection fat. A few pragmatic ways you can consume midsection fat is by following a solid eating routine and ordinary activity. Additionally, spices like ginger, lemon, cumin, green tea, and bean stew pepper could assist you with diminishing the fat substance in your body.

You can likewise counsel your PCP on the off chance that the home cures are not working out and the fat aggregation influences your well-being. Connect with your primary care physician and get the vital well-being exhortation.

Chapter 4

Exercise and Weight Reduction

The Significance of Weight Reduction and Exercise

Weight can prompt various serious medical issues, including coronary illness, diabetes, stroke, and a few sorts of diseases.

One technique that can assist an individual with shedding pounds is to restrict the quantity of calories taken in through their eating regimen. The alternate way is to consume additional calories while working out.

Benefits of Exercise vs. Diet

Joining exercise with a sound eating routine is a more powerful method for getting in shape than contingent upon calorie limitation alone. Exercise can forestall or try to oppose the impacts of specific infections. Practice brings down pulse and cholesterol, which might forestall coronary failure.

Moreover, if you work out, you bring down your gamble of fostering specific kinds of tumors like colon and bosom disease. Practice is likewise known to help add to a feeling of certainty and prosperity, consequently conceivably bringing down paces of uneasiness and sadness.

Practice is useful for weight reduction and keeping up with weight reduction. Exercise can build digestion, or the number of calories you consume in a day. It can likewise help you keep up with and increment lean weight, which additionally assists increment with the numbering of calories you consume every day.

What amount of Exercise Is Required for Weight reduction?

To receive the well-being rewards of activity, it is prescribed that you play out some type of vigorous activity no less than three times each week for at least 20 minutes for every meeting. Nonetheless, over 20 minutes is better if you need to get in shape. Consolidating only 15 minutes of moderate activity, for example, strolling one mile consistently will wreck to an additional 100 calories (accepting you don't consume an abundance of calories in your eating routine thereafter). Consuming 700 calories in seven days can approach 10 lbs. of weight reduction throughout the year.

Calculating Your Target Heart Rate

To get all of the medical advantages of activity, you'll have to blend in some higher power works out. To find out about how hard you are functioning, you can check your pulse. The essential equation for deciding your objective pulse is to take away your age from 220 and afterwards ascertain 60 to 80 percent of that number.

Converse with a mentor or your medical care group to assist you with deciding your best power for every exercise. Those with unique well-being concerns like a physical issue, diabetes, or a heart condition ought to counsel a doctor before starting any workout schedule.

Few Instances of the Various Sorts of Activity?

The sort of activity you decide for weight reduction doesn't make any difference however much whether you're getting it done. That is the reason specialists suggest you pick practices you appreciate so that you'll adhere to a customary daily schedule.

Aerobic

Regardless of what exercise program you execute, it ought to incorporate some type of vigorous or cardiovascular activity. aerobic activities get your pulse up and your blood siphoning. Aerobic activities might incorporate strolling, running, cycling, swimming, and moving. You can likewise sort it out on a wellness machine like a treadmill, curved, or step stepper.

Cardio exercise and weight

One of the most famous kinds of activity for weight reduction is a high-impact workout, otherwise called cardio. Models include:

• strolling

• running

• cycling

• swimming

Aerobic activity doesn't significantly affect your bulk, basically not contrasted with lifting loads. Nonetheless, it is exceptionally successful at consuming calories.

A 10-month concentrate inspected how cardio without eating fewer carbs impacted 141 individuals with heftiness or overweight. Members were parted into three gatherings and not told to lessen calorie admission.

The individuals who consumed 400 calories for every cardio meeting (5 times each week) lost 4.3% of their body weight, while the people who consumed 600 calories for every meeting (likewise 5 times each week) lost somewhat more, at 5.7%. The benchmark group, which didn't work out, really put on 0.5% of their body weight.

Different examinations likewise show that cardio can assist you with consuming fat, particularly the hazardous stomach fat that expands your gamble of type 2 diabetes and coronary illness.

That implies adding cardio to your way of life is probably going to assist you with dealing with your weight and work on your metabolic well-being, assuming you keep your caloric intake the same.

Weight Training

A major benefit of working out with loads is that as well as shedding fat, you'll fabricate muscle. Muscle, thus, consumes calories. Discuss a sound criticism circle! Specialists suggest working all the significant muscle bunches three times each week. This incorporates:

• abs

• back

• biceps

- calves

- chest

- lower arms

- hamstrings

- quads

- shoulders

- traps

- rear arm muscles

Yoga

Yoga isn't quite as extraordinary as different kinds of activity, however, it can assist you with shedding pounds in alternate ways, as per a new report by scientists. The investigation discovered that individuals who practice yoga are more careful about what they eat and, in this way, less inclined to have stoutness.

Integrating Activity Into Your Way of Life

The aggregate sum of activity you take part in during a day matters more than whether you do it in a solitary meeting. That is the reason little changes in your everyday schedule can have a major effect on your waistline.

A solid way of life propensities to consider include:

• strolling or riding your bicycle to work or while getting things done

• using the stairwell rather than the lift

• stopping farther away from objections and strolling the leftover distance

Exercises and How Much Calories They Consume

The typical grown-up male who doesn't practice requires roughly 2,200 calories every day to keep up with his typical weight. A female necessities around 1,800 calories to keep up with her weight.

The accompanying rundown contains normal exercises and the surmised measure of calories consumed each hour:

Exercises

Calories Consumed

playing baseball, golf, or cleaning the house

240 to 300

lively strolling, trekking, moving, or planting

370 to 460

playing football, running (at a nine-minute-mile speed), or swimming

580 to 730

skiing, racquetball, or running (at a seven-minute-mile pace)

740 to 920

0 seconds of 0 seconds

Before You Start an Activity Program

Converse with your primary care physician before you start another activity program, particularly assuming you are anticipating doing incredible activity. This is particularly significant assuming you have:

• coronary illness

• lung infection

• diabetes

• kidney infection

• joint pain

Individuals who have been exceptionally latent for the new months, who are overweight, or have as of late stopped smoking ought to likewise converse with their PCPs before starting another activity program.

At the point when you are initially beginning another activity program, it's vital to focus on the signs your body is giving you. You ought to propel yourself, with the goal that your wellness level moves along. Be that as it may, propelling yourself too hard can make you harm yourself. Quit practicing on the off chance that you begin to encounter agony or windedness.

Practicing has many advantages. Opposition preparation can assist with weight reduction by keeping up with bulk and supporting digestion. Cardio can likewise help yet may make you hungrier, so attempt to carefully eat.

If you're attempting to get thinner, you might be considering the amount you ought to exercise and what sorts of activity you ought to do.

At its easiest, getting thinner means consuming a larger number of calories than you consume. Along these lines, it's a good idea to remember practice for your daily schedule, since it assists you with consuming more calories.

Be that as it may, enthusiastic activity can likewise assist you with burning some serious calories. This might create turmoil about the job of practice in weight reduction and whether it can help.

All in all, what precisely is the reason for practice assuming you're attempting to get more fit? This article investigates the proof to assist you with finding the response and sorting out what's best for you.

Strength exercise and weight

All active work can assist you with consuming calories.

Nonetheless, obstruction preparation, for example, powerlifting has benefits that go past that. Obstruction preparation helps increment the strength, tone, and measure of muscle you have.

One investigation of 141 more seasoned grown-ups with heftiness inspected the impacts of cardio, opposition preparing, or both on body structure during a time of purposeful weight reduction. This investigation discovered that the people who did no activity or cardio alone lost fat yet additionally lost more muscle and bone mass than the gatherings who did obstruction preparation.

In this way, obstruction preparation seems to defensively affect both muscle and bone during times of diminished calorie consumption.

Higher measures of muscle likewise increment your digestion, assisting you with consuming more calories nonstop even very still. This is because muscle is more metabolically dynamic than fat, meaning it requires more energy.

This likewise forestalls the drop in digestion that can happen close to weight reduction.

Along these lines, doing some type of obstruction preparation is a pivotal expansion to a viable long-haul weight reduction plan. It makes it more straightforward to keep the load off, which is a lot harder than losing it in any case.

Extreme cardio exercise and weight

Extreme cardio exercise (HIIT) is a sort of activity portrayed by short explosions of extraordinary activity followed by a concise rest before rehashing this cycle. HIIT should be possible with cardio or obstruction preparing practices and gives the advantages of both.

Most HIIT exercises are just 10-20 minutes in length, however, they offer strong advantages as to weight reduction.

One 2017 survey of 13 great investigations discovered that HIIT and cardio practice gave comparable advantages specifically, decreased muscle versus fat and midsection boundary for individuals with overweight and heftiness.

Nonetheless, HIIT practice accomplished these equivalent advantages with a 40% time investment fund contrasted with cardio.

As a result of the power of HIIT, you ought to counsel a medical care professional before beginning another HIIT schedule, particularly if you have realized heart concerns.

Exercise and hunger

You've presumably heard that actual effort is an effective method for burning some serious calories, or perhaps you even ended up eating more than expected after an enthusiastic exercise.

Notwithstanding, most exploration focuses on practice having a hunger concealment impact.

One concentrate in 20 dynamic, solid grown-ups noticed that they ate more food in the feast before an exercise than later and really viewed that as, generally speaking, members ate less food when they practiced than the days they didn't.

In one more concentrate on 26 ladies with heftiness on low-calorie eats, scientists found that short HIIT meetings had areas of strength for a stifling impact.

Scientists have likewise noticed that morning exercise seems, by all accounts, to be more valuable for energy equilibrium and calorie admission than night practice further supporting the hypothesis that exercise can lessen craving.

In any case, more examination is required, and hunger reactions to practice are probable exceptionally person. On the off chance that you're attempting to get thinner but will generally eat more than expected after enthusiastic or long activity meetings, think about more limited spans (like HIIT) or less extraordinary activity.

Different advantages of activity

Practice is truly perfect for your well-being in numerous ways, not simply concerning weight on the board.

Ordinary activity can further develop your glucose control and may assist with lessening your gamble of ongoing infections like coronary illness, type 2 diabetes, and certain malignant growths.

Practice additionally assists you with keeping up with and developing your bulk, keeping your bones solid and thick, and forestalling the beginning of conditions like osteoporosis which is portrayed by bone fragility.

Also, practice offers a few mental advantages. It can assist you with diminishing your feelings of anxiety and overseeing pressure all the more actually, and it seems to offer some assurance against neurodegenerative circumstances like Alzheimer's illness.

Remember these advantages when you think about the impacts of activity. Regardless of whether it significantly impacts weight reduction, it has different advantages that are similarly as though (not more) significant.

Proposals

Given its various medical advantages, exercise ought to be a piece of your routine no matter what your weight objectives.

Truth be told, the best weight reduction maintainers recorded in the Public Weight Control Vault, who have lost something like 30 pounds (14 kg) and kept it off for somewhere around 1 year, report practicing for no less than 1 hour out of each day.

The Actual Work Rules for Americans frame ideal activity sums for all ages to assist with advancing well-being. For grown-ups, they are:

• Oxygen-consuming (cardio) workout: 150-300 moderate power minutes or 75-150 energetic force minutes out of each week

• Muscle-fortifying (opposition) workout: at least 2 days out of every seven days of activities using all significant muscle gatherings

Notwithstanding, on the off chance that your objective is weight reduction, you ought to focus on diet over practice since it will have a lot bigger effect. On the off chance that your time is restricted, consider obstruction preparation (as opposed to cardio) to assist with keeping up with your bulk and metabolic rate or HIIT to assist you with accomplishing a comparable calorie consumption as cardio significantly quicker.

Moreover, don't rely just on the scale to keep tabs on your development. If you are acquiring muscle while losing fat, your weight may not change as fast as you'd like it to — in any case, you'll be better for it. Think about accepting your estimations too, and monitor how your garments fit. These are vastly improved marks of fat misfortune than weight alone.

The reality

Practice is significant for general well-being, and various kinds of activity might offer various benefits for weight reduction.

If you're attempting to get in shape, you may be especially keen on opposition preparation, which can safeguard your sans-fat mass and increment your calories consumed very still, and HIIT, which gives similar advantages as cardio, however for less time.

However, recall, with an objective of practical weight reduction, it's likewise truly vital to follow an unobtrusive calorie-limited diet contained generally of entire food sources.